Included:

The Exhibitionist's Game
    An explanation of the game, where the idea came from and examples from some who have tried it

The Rubber Band Trick
    Also some tricks and tips for breast/nipple play

Story: The Chase

Orgasm Roulette
    Orgasm after orgasm after orgasm...

Story: How To Train Your Vagina… To Whistle

The Exhibitionist's Game

Send nudes.

Okay, okay. The game is WAY more complicated than that. And, it's a lot more fun than simply exchanging dick and pussy pics. It can be a lot of fun, but also deeply satisfying and even has some good learning about self that can enhance your personal sexuality. I dare say it might even be able to boost self esteem and improve overall enjoyment of life.

Can a fun, online exchange do all that? Sure. Send nudes.

No, no. I'm just kidding. There's a lot to figure out before we get to that.

Imagine a line with Voyeur at one end and Exhibitionist at the other. We ALL fit somewhere on that line. WHY we are where we are and the rewards we are seeking are all very personal. But, we are all somewhere along that line.

For some, the reward is feeling dirty and slutty. For others, there is freedom to exhibiting themselves. Some may enjoy the adrenaline rush of showing off to a stranger. Another person may enjoy showing off ONLY to their partner, but in a place or setting that has some risk to it. There are literally thousands of reasons to get off on showing off.

Starting out, you may think you are HERE on that line and you may think you know why you are THERE. The game though, is to have some fun exploring and challenging yourself.

Before you begin the game, you'll need to establish what you think about yourself and why you like this. That means A LOT of conversation between you and your chosen voyeur to figure all that out and make sure that both of you understand where you think you are on the line. With any luck, you'll learn something new about yourself and your exhibitionist desires.

Step 1:
Find The Right Play Partner

If you are an exhibitionist, you have to find yourself a voyeur to play with. Someone that will enjoy receiving your pics, of course. BUT, this is not about exchanging nude pics. It's about the challenge. So, your voyeur needs to be someone who understands your specific needs and goals with exhibitionism and can push you to expand and explore those needs and goals.

Your voyeur also has to be rewarded. If they just want nudes, they can go online and see all they want. Don't take that personal. No matter how hot you may be, the internet is full of hot naked folks.

The rewards for this game are cerebral and have to be satisfying on a mental level or it gets very boring, very fast. Being a voyeur can be just as individual as the exhibitionist. So, you need to find a match that compliments your game, not just your naked ass.

As an example, I am all voyeur. I have an impressive resume of photography. I am an artist. I am going to be FAR less interested in seeing one more naked woman but much more interested in seeing a naked women who can be very creative with her selfies. I want to see good composition and interesting color, not just "Is my pussy pretty?"

As that intelligent voyeur, I am going to be less interested in the blatantly sexual nature of a photo, or how many different places you can get blurry cell phone shots of your pooper and more interested in how original you can be when you flash that pooper as well as the quality of the art itself.

If you just want to send nudes and hear that you're pretty, I would be a terrible voyeur for you to play this game with. I don't need spank material; I want some THINK material. Challenging you on a cerebral level is what this game is about. If you are looking for validation, or want to exorcise some childhood demons, you need to find a voyeur that matches you well with that. If you want to shock people with random incidents of flashing, find a voyeur that will compliment that aspect.

For me, I also want a story, being a storyteller myself. Every picture tells a story and I want the pics I receive to have a story to them in some way. Or, I want them to be like chapters of a larger story you're telling. That's just me, though.

I also think the game has to have a progression or it will get boring. Each picture needs to be going somewhere. That's just me. Your story is yours though. How you tell it is yours. How you play is up to you. So, find a voyeur that matches how you want to play.

Step 2:
Establish A Point System

Your game doesn't necessarily have to have points, literally, but it helps to build something towards a reward of some kind. After 50 points, for example, you get a reward. Your point system can be anything and you can establish it any way you want. But, each pic you send your voyeur has to get graded or judged in some way. Did it meet the goals of the pic? How did it build towards the end goal? Did it challenge you in some way? How well did the pic tell your story?

Just another nude? Low points because I fell asleep. A nude standing next to a nun who is unaware of your nakedness? High points. Well, if that is how you and your voyeur are playing it would be. The point system is between you and your voyeur to decide on.

While exhibitionism generally means NUDE pics, it doesn't necessarily need to be. The pics can include some sort of risk or maybe something that is out of the camera view. You and your voyeur can decide the content. There's an example of this below.

The voyeur decides the value of each pic. The voyeur's decision is final, although you may plead your case for a better score. Since you have no decision in the points, it is up to you to push yourself a little to try to get more points. You keep sending the same pic, you won't earn many points. Send a pic that is challenging, you'll get more points. Since you don't know what grade your voyeur will give you, you will be motivated to work a little harder each pic.

Step 3:
Figure Out A Reward System

Being miles apart, and/or not being play partners, how shall your voyeur reward you? Or, punish you? Giving you a "good girl" for every pic will get so boring. Slash my wrists sort of boring. As you build points, it has to be TOWARDS something.

It could be similar to the D/s relationship if that works for you. You earn rewards, or you get punished depending on the system you and your voyeur agree to. Setting up a point system is vital. Figuring out your rewards for points earned is vital-er. Without it, the game gets boring fast and goes nowhere. If this game isn't moving forward at all times, it will quickly grind to a halt.

Actual financial rewards where your voyeur is sending you money or gifts defeats the purpose of the game. In that case, your voyeur is basically paying you for your nude pics. Boring. There's no challenge in that. And, as soon as your voyeur discovers the internet, the game will end.

Unless you are partners or live close by, the game has to be entirely on the honor system. There's no real way to enforce punishment or deliver rewards long distance (except for money, but see above). Your voyeur just has to trust that you're not cheating on your rewards. I will add that cheating will be very unsatisfying for you and it will get boring for your voyeur. For the game to continue and be fun, each has to have some trust that they're both playing honorably.

Step 4:
The Goal Line

In chess, the game ends when you capture the king. This game needs a goal like that. That way, you and your voyeur can gauge progress of your exploration and how close you are to achieving your goals. The game will get boring if it just goes on and on with no marks to shoot for. You can always start a new game after the first one. But, each stage of the game needs a goal line of some sort.

Without this step, the game is truly pointless and is nothing more than sending nudes. Ugh!!

Your game, your rules. Use the four steps as a guide and it will be fun and challenging. That's so much better than just sending nudes. Right?

Keep in mind that women flashing men can easily be misinterpreted, so keep a security plan in mind for any men who get aggressive.

My only other cautions are to be aware of kids and pets that might be present.

And don't do anything that will put you in the hospital or jail. From the arresting officer to the sentencing judge, the legal folks do not usually see the fun in this game. Other than that, go be adventurous and have fun!!

The Original Source
Of This Game

Sigh. What prompted this post is a conversation with a woman named Carly who might play the game with me. She loves the freedom of nakedness. She loves the artistry of the human body. She is attracted to the unusual scenarios of being naked in public, not the inappropriateness. She says she loves attention, but getting the attention really isn't about sex. It's kinda like a "free the nipple" type thing.

So, I've asked her to pick out an outfit that is easy to change into and then, when the photo op arises, she can strip out of quickly for her pic. Then after, she can redress just as quickly for her escape. Since I love a good story and she appreciates the storytelling angle, I have a game planned out that I think she'll enjoy and we'll have a lot of fun with. An outfit she can get in and out of quickly will be instrumental in her success.

I'm going to have her tell me a story about her town - which turns out to be a very small town. She will be the town's Naked Tourism Ambassador. Twelve photos in twelve locations with twelve stories. All naked. Imagine ME as a prospective vacationer and she has to sell me on taking my vacation to her town. With each photo she'll need to send me 2-3 sentences about the location, telling me what makes that location so interesting.

For each completed photo, Carly gets 10 points. If she's only topless or bottomless, she gets 5 points. No story, she loses 3 points. The photo MUST show that she is naked. When she reaches 150 points, she gets her reward.

Um… If you do the math, 12 photos worth 10 points each only adds up to 120. True. So I gave her the ability to score extra credit, so she can reach the necessary 150 points.

First, throw in some interesting trivia and earn an extra point or two. Ho hum.

Throw in some extra naked people and earn 10 points each. The people have to be strangers that she dragged into the scene on location. Women can be topless or bottomless for 5 points. Totally naked for 10 points. Men have to be totally naked because topless men is too easy. She can enlist friends, but friends are only worth 5 points at best, if they're totally naked. Bringing a friend that she talked into this project is like low hanging fruit. A friend that is only topless or bottomless is only worth 2 points.

Should she accomplish her goal of 150 points, I owe her a reward. What I decided on was to use my wealth of experience as a graphic designer and put together a mock tourism brochure of her photos and information that she can post or print. How cool would that be?!?! This should be fun. Update to come.

Update: Carly completed her goal of the 12 photos with ease in about 30 days. Each photo was accompanied by a little story about why she chose that location and why it's an interesting site in her town. She also threw in little bits of town history and trivia to gain a few extra points.

She earned some of the extra points needed by talking 8 members of a road construction crew - men AND women - to drop their pants and moon the camera with her. It was accompanied by a wonderfully creative caption about the endless road construction in town.

She also earned bonus points after enlisting a sidekick. The manager of a very popular fast food restaurant caught her taking a pic in the drive thru and instead of calling the cops, she asked to join in. She wasn't as bold as Carly, but she turned out to be a great storyteller and was able to help with location ideas. And, she was a nice addition to the single subject pics in the few pics that she was in.

Finally, she got the last of her extra points by touring a grocery store and getting women in the store to flash their breasts while holding up various items in the store, Vanna White style. Those photos had captions bragging about how much fun it is to go shopping at that store, which had been in the same location since right after the civil war.

The final achievement was when she confessed that her MOM was in one of the photos!!

A Few Game Examples:

Janice

A woman I played this game with a few years ago was terribly aroused by the danger of showing off in public, but never had the courage to go through with it. So, the goal for her was to increase the number of people and the risk involved. When she scored enough points, she got to walk down a particular busy street completely naked, which was a HUGE fantasy of hers.

The pics leading up to that, increased her courage to build up to it. First photo was to flash one boob at a single stranger. Each photo after, more people and more naked for a longer amount of time. We estimated that her walk would last about 15 minutes before it got too risky and there would be about 250 people on the street and in the businesses along the street that might see her. It took about 6 months to work up to it.

She found it exhilarating for her personally. It gave her courage to make changes in her life that she wanted. Career and relationships all took a step up. She took a vacation to Europe. She stopped living cautiously because of the risks in life and started living courageously in spite of them.

PS. Yes, we planned the timing of her walk for 11:00 pm, and it was in an area where there were unlikely to be any children. Most people probably thought she was drunk, which was fine. Most gawked. A few hollered distasteful comments. But, no one bothered her and she got to complete her walk to a waiting car.

Angie & Mark

Another woman, who played the game with her husband, was into strangers seeing her discreetly. The rule was, no sex until she had shown off to a set number of strangers. When she reached her goal, he'd fuck her silly. But until then… Nothing. She wasn't even allowed to masturbate.

Each time they restarted the game, they picked a different group of strangers or a different setting. One time, it was strangers on the subway. Another time, it was in the grocery store!! Each time, it was different. And each time they restarted, they tried to find a more challenging group to flash.

Don't misunderstand. He LOVED fucking his wife. But making her wait, and him waiting, made things so much hotter when they finally got together.

Lillith

My favorite, an art student I knew, got very creative. She set her camera up in a little cafe in the old city (Knoxville). She sat at a table in the front window drinking coffee and eating lunch. The camera was on the bar sort of behind her. She was wearing a skirt and nothing underneath. She set the camera for the self timer to shoot a pic every 30 seconds. No one in the cafe could see what she was doing. But, people passing by on the street could see her lift her skirt and flash her goods.

The pics she sent me (6 total) didn't show me anything except the facial expressions of people passing by and catching a glimpse under her skirt. Most of those were slightly blurred because they were moving. But, I could see them well enough. There were five men and one older woman who was smiling from ear to ear - and staring!

She said her camera ran out of memory at about 40 pics, and most pics didn't catch anyone seeing her. But... The ones she caught were priceless!! She also said she flashed dozens of other people, but it wasn't timed with the camera taking the photo.

I didn't actually see any of her bits from the camera angle. I still gave her double points for all the preparation this took and for her creativity.

Next, she took a series of photos using the glass to reflect her beautiful girl parts back to the camera. The glass for that series was a window inside a store at the mall and all kinds of people could see her if they looked her direction. Not sure anyone did. It still took some creativity to get the lighting and camera angle right.

And, it took some serious bravado to go through with it.

Lee & Sarah

Another woman I talked to played this game with her partner. They had both lost weight and loved their new bodies. However, the weight loss, kids, age and miles had given them saggy, deflated breasts they hated.

Their challenge was that they had to somehow sneak a photo of themselves topless next to the sign for each of the 33 doctors in their area that did breast augmentation surgery. They had to be very creative with that since some of the signs were right out on the street. Other signs were inside buildings and were VERY public.

Once they had a photo of the sign, they were allowed to call that particular doctor and ask for information. When they had photos with the signs of all 33, they were allowed to go in for a consult to any of the doctors they liked.

The way they announced to each other which doctor they had chosen was to go back and get another topless pic WITH that doctor. And once they did that, they were able to set an appointment and get the work done.

Julia & Tom

There was also the couple that were huge baseball fans. She had to flash her breasts at every ball park in the Major Leagues and get a selfie in the stands without getting thrown out.

It was tricky - more so than you might think. She got thrown out of several games. Her husband played dumb and acted like he knew nothing about it, even as he was being thrown out right along with her. LOL.

When they had been to every ball park, they bought themselves tickets to the World Series.

Ben & Allie

Another couple, both exhibitionists and voyeurs right in the middle of that line, sorta played "H-O-R-S-E". She'd display herself in some way, send him the pic. He'd have to match it. Not only the pic, but the location and pose as closely as possible.

Male and female, there are some pics more "do-able" for each. They each started with 10 points. For each pic that wasn't duplicated, that person lost a point. Whoever ran out of points first, had to pay for their next night out and the person who still had points could choose any night out they wanted. Dinner, movie, ballet, art shows. One time they went to some kind of a farming fair thing (LOL). Whatever the winner wanted and the loser had to pay for it with a smile.

The nice things about their game was that it never had an end. They just restarted and kept going after someone won.

Fran

A woman I told about this game had a unique situation. She worked for a large department store in NYC. She had a serious crush on the guy who did the store windows. He did some beautiful and elaborate window designs - even won awards for them.

She would sneak in and "photobomb" his pics of the windows. He's outside in the street with the camera, and by the time her got in to get mad at her, she would be gone, hiding within the store.

Her hope was to be right in the front of the window and for him to photograph her in plain view of everyone. Usually though, she was back a little so she could sneak in and out quickly. This wasn't actually a game, but maybe will give you ideas.

Eventually she let him catch her and they lived happily ever after.

Joey & Clark

One set of partners required that the exhibitionist was to put a penny in two jars for each photo. The jars sat on an old scales of justice. Some points were positive and went into one jar; some points were negative and went into the other jar. The end was like reward and/or punishment depending on which jar bottomed out first. They were very creative.

The first month, if her positive jar filled first, she got to watch TV on the nice 48" TV with the great sound system. If the negative jar filled first, she had to watch TV on an old BW 13" TV.

Second month, positive meant she could drink any wine she wanted. Negative meant she could only drink beer (which she apparently didn't like).

Like Ben & Allie, this game never had to end. They could just restart it with new rewards and punishments each time.

The Rubber Band Trick

1) Make sure the areole and nipple is very dry. Wet nipples will cause the rubber band to slip off.

2) Wrap a rubber band around the nipple. Tight enough that it will securely stay in place, but not so tight it will cut off circulation.

   * Some experimentation may be necessary to find the right size rubber band that will attach securely. Small nipples may require smaller rubber bands. But, smaller thickness of rubber bands can cause cutting into the tissue or limiting circulation.

3) Put the other end of the rubber band in her teeth. Some experimentation may be needed to find the right length of rubber bands so that the rubber band is stretched very tight between nipple and teeth.

4) Commence goal oriented play, attempting to bring her to orgasm quickly.

One of two things will happen. Either she will "forget" that the rubber band is there and open her mouth to breathe harder, and "SNAP!!", which will deliver a small rush of endorphins, slightly intensifying her orgasm. If she enjoys a little pain with her pleasure, even better.

Or, she will not be able to forget the rubber band is there and what will happen if she does, and she will be so distracted that it keeps her on the edge, which will also intensify the orgasm (when she finally cums).

An escalation of this game, or for those of you who are into breast binding or breasts torture of some kind. BTW, let me say that strict binding and torture of the breasts can have serious consequences. I cannot recommend against it enough.

That said, a reasonably safe way to bind the breasts without ropes is with a condom. Cut the tip off and stretch it open. Slide it over the breast all the way with just the nipple exposed. It constricts enough to get the sensation without causing serious circulation issues. The constriction will cause the nipple to get WAY more sensitive, for the rubber band trick, or for ANY kind of nipple stimulation.

I know a woman who has used this trick to increase the amount of milk that she shoots from her breasts in her ANR. It doesn't seem to increase milk production. It just squeezes the breasts in an efficient manner for releasing that milk. Just letting you know, for those into that.

Note: Small nipples might need to be pumped until they are full enough or long enough to attach the rubber band. Pumping brings more blood into the nipple, which may intensify the sensations even more. Make sure to dry them fully before attempting to attach the rubber band.

Note: This same trick can be used on the clit on some women. Pumping may be necessary to increase the size of the clit enough to attach the rubber band. Make sure the tissue is dry when attempting to attach. You may need to knot two or more rubber bands together to stretch far enough. Also, body position should be so that the rubber band is unobstructed from teeth to clit. This is easiest achieved in piledriver position. Tie her legs up over her head and you should have no problems.

Back to the condom as a binding technique. There are actually several uses for this that can be lots of fun. As stated above, it increases the sensitivity of the nipples by constricting the remaining breast. Imagine having an orgasm simply by touching the nipples gently and lightly. This is MY personal favorite. Some women have very sensitive breasts and nipples without enhancing them in any way. Many, many women can have orgasms from breast or nipple stimulation.

For others, it is quite the opposite. There is very little sensitivity. Or, the sensitivity they experience is unlikely to cause an orgasm. Orgasm is very much about the mental association to the stimulation. It is also possible, they have never associated orgasm to their breasts. This type of breasts play can increase sensitivity enough to make that leap. And then, even without the binding, they are able to experience breast-gasms or nipple-gasms. YAY!!

Applying the condoms on other parts of the body might be difficult. But apply the thinking. It is conceivable that stimulation of ANY part of a woman's body can lead to orgasm. Experiment and find ways to stimulate any part of her body that interests you. By using your energy to connect, by gently and patiently exploring, you may find a plethora of ways to experience pleasure together.

Story: The Chase

The chase ends immediately upon capture of the prey.

It also ends if the prey escapes.

If it is the chase that excites you, then you must guarantee that neither conclusion is achieved.

Stalking** is the deciding factor. If you stalk well, quietly, discretely, then the capture is certain. If you are clumsy or unintelligent, then you will alert your prey. It will startle and escape, usually before the chase really begins. Therefore, the stalking is the means by which the end is achieved. So to perpetuate the chase, stalking is out. To perpetuate the chase, you must carefully chase (or be chased) and do so until you are ready for the chase to end.

Sometimes, seduction takes years. Long, beautiful, wonderful years before it reaches its conclusion - either one. Seduction is a dance, not a race. If the dance is what excites you (as prey or predator), and the capture is just the beginning of the boredom that comes quickly without the chase, you must keep every step at a distance that is just inside of absolute safety. Safety is boring.

"If I actually wanted to be caught, I wouldn't run," she says.

"If I actually wanted to catch her, I would run faster," he says.

Neither is happy when the chase ends. Therefore, the seduction continues.

A few years ago, I talked to a very wealthy couple in their 70s. I had actually met them years before when they were about 60. I challenged them to continue looking for adventure. Always.

They had retired from very successful careers. They had raised several children and grandchildren. They had traveled the country and the globe, not just as tourists, but as adventurers. "So, what do you do now?" I asked them.

"Sometimes, we play strip hide and seek," she told me. "Every time we find each other, they have to take something off."

"Sometimes," he snickered, "I'll hide and take off everything but my socks."

I got this mental image of her opening a pantry door and her naked husband jumping out, scaring her to death.

She laughed at him. "That would be a good strategy if you hid in a place I could find you. You always find the craziest places in the house to hide."

They had a VERY large house. It had LOTS of crazy places to hide.

"Other times, he just chases me around the house."

He grinned. "That's my favorite, I think."

"He'll chase me and chase me, both of us laughing like crazy people, until we're too tired to do anything but just lay there and hold hands." She turned to him and smiled. "I think that's my favorite too."

** Not that kind of stalking. One is a heinous, criminal act. The other, as referred to here, is a balance of seduction between predator and prey.

Orgasm Roulette

I want to preface this by saying that ALL women are not good candidates for this game. I am confident that all women CAN accomplish this, but not all women WILL let go as fully as this game requires. They can learn. And if she's willing to learn, this game is an awesome tool to get there. If she's already "orgasm roulette ready", this game delivers an endless stream of orgasms.

Fair warning though, that many orgasms back-to-back-to-back can be a bit overwhelming for some women. Fun, but a bit overwhelming. If your sub is a masochist, this can be a fun bit of torture (although it rarely causes pain). If you're a sadist and your sub is okay with that… Well, go have fun.

She needs to be a fairly orgasmic woman and it works best if she is naturally submissive to her Dom. It might be fun if you're just roleplaying. But for best results, the energy has to be natural. I guess that could be said for almost anything. Hmmm… A sex game as a metaphor for life. Sure!!

In the best scenario, she is a woman who has experience with having anal orgasms as well as orgasms from vaginal or clitoral stimulation, AND, this is even better if she has some experience with throatgasms. If she has not had a lot of experience with any of these, this is a game that might improve that.

Ladies, I will also add that this game can be modified to suit your level of being able to trust and let go, or your level of training if you're using this to learn some new tricks. Really, this game can probably be modified to suit any couple's interests and abilities.

Women can have so many different types of orgasms that I am actually jealous. When I have played this game with previous partners, I admit, my female side was kinda living vicariously though them. Sigh.

To play the game as I'll detail it (and again, you can modify this to suit your own variation, but this is how I play it), you'll need:

* several pillows that can be thrown on the floor or carpet for her to kneel on for the final stage of play

* I also recommend puppy pads spread generously on the pillows in case she squirts (grins)

* You'll need a vibrating butt plug or a vibrating dildo of some kind that is large enough to give her a "full" feeling, but not so big that the stretching is a distraction. The main thing is that it needs to stay in place when she starts having back to back orgasms.

* A Hitachi or similar heavy duty vibrator - even better if she is familiar with it and has been successful using it prior to this.

Ready to play? Let's go!!

Take off all your clothes and have the woman lay on the bed, on her back. Start with some kissing and touching as foreplay.

Go down on her or use the Hitachi and bring her to an orgasm or two. You don't want to dwell on it. The idea is simply to "prime the pump" and get her going.

Next, flip her over and eat her ass like you're trying to win a prize at the state fair. I mean, really eat her passionately. Get her ass so horny that she almost can't control herself. If she cums, awesome!! That would be the goal. But eventually, you're going to insert the aforementioned toy into her and you want it to be orgasmic.

Once she's good and warmed up, hopefully an anal orgasm or two, insert the anal plug to keep things warm.

Now, move to the pillows. Have her kneel, lowering herself on to the head of the Hitachi, which is laying on the pillows and puppy pads. Make sure she is low enough that she can easily move her hips to press her clit on the Hitachi AND can move her hips back to add pressure from the anal plug.

Sometimes, it is helpful to restrain her hands behind her back, but that depends on the woman and the energy between the two of you. Some like that and it helps; others not so much. Restrained or not, she is not to use her hands for any of this.

Once she is in position, stand in front of her and present your penis for her mouth. SLOWLY begin to fuck her mouth. The deeper, the better. But, you're not trying to choke her or cause asphyxiation. Starting out, you want this to be slow and gentle. Focus on this until she has an oral / throat orgasm. Repeat a couple of times.

And then the fun REALLY begins.

Once she has had a throatgasm or two, begin to gradually increase the tempo and intensity. You're never going to escalate to the point of actually throatfucking her in the brutal, stereotypical definition. Just fast and hard enough that it is difficult to focus on anything else but breathing.

Breathing is very important.

As you fuck her mouth, suddenly instruct her, "Pussy!", indicating for her to have a vaginal orgasm, rubbing her clit against the Hitachi.

As she levels off, shove yourself balls deep in her mouth and instruct her, "Throat!", indicating for her to have another throatgasm. Be aware that breathing will be compromised and you'll need to adjust yourself in her throat accordingly.

As she levels off, instruct her, "Ass!", indicating for her to have an anal orgasm.

And then instruct her, "Pussy!"

Or, "Throat!"

Or, "Ass!"

Your choice. Sometimes, you can call for "Pussy!" three times in a row. Sometimes, you can spread the timing out to an excruciating pace to tease her. Change up the order so she doesn't know what's next.

Starting out, let her recover a little before you instruct her to have the next orgasm. But gradually, as you get closer to your own orgasm, increase the speed until she is literally having one orgasm after another.

When it's time for you to shoot your load, you want to be telling her, "Throat! Throat! Throat!" because there is nothing as nice as having an orgasm in her throat while SHE has an orgasm in her throat. That's about as good as it gets.

If your girl has never experienced a throatgasm, the energy of this might be the extra spark to get her there. If she has difficulty reaching orgasm of ANY kind, the energy and intensity of this game might help. Same with anal orgasms.

Find the toys that work best for you. Find a "flow" that works best for you. Experiment and adjust this versatile game to suit whatever works best for you. I have a potential candidate that we might have to find a way to include spanking her. Yep, she has "spankgasms". I'm not sure how we'll work that in, but I am excited to figure it out. And you too, might have variations that will be fun to try and include, even if you get it wrong the first few times. Like all games, the biggest goal is to have fun. As long as you're having fun, everybody win.

After she swallows the load in her throat, she may fall over exhausted. It might take her a while to fully catch her breath. Help her pull the plug out of her ass and move cautiously away from the Hitachi. If she wants to just sleep right there on the floor, let her. Don't bother counting the orgasms. Just know by the smile on her face that it was plenty.

Story: How To Train Your Vagina... To Whistle

I was making dinner when the phone rang. I saw the caller ID was from Minnesota and almost didn't answer. But, then I remembered that the ONLY person I know in Minnesota is Brenda and she is always an interesting conversation.

A few years ago, she came to visit me in Knoxville. She originally said she was going to stay two days, but also said she wasn't leaving until she could squirt like Old Faithful. So, I prepared for two days max, being the confident guy that I am.

Usually when someone arrives, we spend the first few hours getting to know each other a little. I'll cook something really good and we'll eat and talk about our goals for their visit. If they've been traveling a long way, they're probably tired. Training of any kind has little chance of success between nervousness at meeting a stranger and the fatigue.

When Brenda arrived though, dinner still had about an hour to simmer. I was making chili and it takes a while to get it just right. So, I suggested we play a little while we waited. Break the ice, so to speak.

"I just came all the way from Minnesota to learn some new tricks. I can eat back home," she said. So, we went into the bedroom.

Forget nerves. Forget any seduction I might have had in mind. Before I could even get a candle lit, she was naked and on the bed.

I laughed. "Horny, much?" I asked her.

When people come to see me, there are two types of visits. Mostly, the reason they are there is to learn something. They aren't necessarily there to play. So even though it is quite sexual in nature, it is almost clinical. Think classroom, not bedroom. Even though I am teaching about their vagina and my fingers are inside them, it is a very different vibe than it probably sounds.

That's one reason that people don't learn much about sex. If you're in bed to play, then play. Have fun. But, if you're there to learn something, you have to keep your eyes on the prize. Once you start playing, the focus often gets lost. One of my greatest responsibilities is to keep the focus on the education.

Women are so much better at that than men. Even though I am rubbing her g-spot and making her cum over and over and over, women can somehow maintain their attention on the lesson. That amazes me. On one hand, they can completely let go and surrender to what's happening. On the other hand, they are learning. Guys are all in one way or the other. And usually, they want to play, which means the lessons get lost.

Brenda and I had not discussed fisting or any kind of actual playing. We had flirted a little on the phone and teased with some playful ideas. She was there to learn to squirt. But all of her pics on FetLife were her vagina stretched wide open with a ginormous toy or a fist in her. That is as good as an invitation for me and I planned on seeing just how much we could stretch her while she was there.

Well, squirting is primarily an exercise of relaxing and just letting go. So, I laid down next to her and began my seduction from there. Some kissing. Some touching. Very gentle stuff as I try to get her to drink the Kool-Aid and relax with me. I am blessed with a very comfortable touch and it's amazing how quickly women surrender when they feel that.

My energy is that I am safe. I am comfortable to relax with. I'm a good human and I can be trusted with their intimacy. It's energy that can be felt. There's no faking it. To have that kind of energy, I have to actually BE that guy. You can't pretend to be safe and trustworthy if you're not. Women can tell.

I can usually feel the moment of surrender. When I kiss her, or touch her or hold her, there is a release in the tension in her body when they feel that energy. That's the moment when the fun begins. Or the lesson. Or both, as Brenda and I had planned.

I was slowly, softly stroking my fingers along her vulva. No rush to push them inside. Just touching. Even on the most outer regions, I could feel some wetness. As I kissed her, I nibbled on her lower lip gently as I slid two fingers into her. They went in so easily, I knew that more was not going to be a problem. It wasn't that she was loose. Not at all. She was plenty tight. Her vagina had perfect flexibility to it. This was a woman who did her Kegels.

"Are you ready to squirt?" I asked her quietly.

Lost in the moment, she only nodded her head submissively. Wanting it, begging in a way. In this case, I used my middle two fingers to quickly brush her g-spot forward. Lightly flicking the pads of my fingertips as fast as I could. It only took about 20 seconds and she made her first mess. She was in heaven and wasn't even aware of it.

I kept brushing her g-spot for about another minute and she continued squirting the whole time. Her face indicated that she was freaking out. Unable to speak, unable to ask what the hell was happening, all she could do was stare into my eyes and continue cumming. Surely she could feel the pool of liquid that was collecting around her ass, which surely added to her freak out.

"Oooohhh mmmyyy G-G-Gooooddd" she eventually managed to get out. I grinned and slid my fingers out of her. Fast and firm, I switched to rubbing her clit back and forth, which launched a new spray of squirt for about 20 seconds. Watching her face, I tried to gauge her threshold. When I thought she needed a break, I stopped and cupped my hand over her entire vulva to let her catch her breath.

As she laid there, I could smell the chili from the kitchen. But, I knew we still had about 20-30 minutes before it was ready. And even then, it wouldn't hurt the chili to simmer a little longer. It was on low. It would be fine.

I rolled over and dug some lube out of the nightstand. I usually go for the expensive natural stuff. I often use coconut oil too. Warmed to a liquid, it is oh so nice. Give it a few seconds in a warm hand and it melts down to the perfect texture.

I positioned myself between her legs and began flicking my tongue across her pussy. Across her labia, inner and outer, across the hood of her clit, across the hole. All over, up and down. She gasped and moaned. I positioned my hands on both sides of her vulva and pushed it together gently. Slowly, I licked up and down. When I let go with my hands, I dove my tongue into the hole and fucked her a few seconds.

When I felt she was ready for the next step, I used my upper lip to push the hood back and began slowly, gently licking back and forth across her exposed clit. That only took a minute or two before she came again.

I sat up onto my knees and got the lube. Her eyes met mine and she knew what was coming. She watched me intently as I slathered the coconut oil all over my right hand. Two fingers first, I flicked them across her g-spot again, causing another orgasm. As she came, I went for it. I closed my hand and shoved it all the way inside.

Instantly, she froze. Her moan was so loud the neighbors probably got turned on. Slowly at first, I worked in and out, gradually building tempo. "Yes, yes, yes," she whispered. Soon, I was halfway to my elbow as I went in, amazed at the depth she was able to take.

After she came a couple of times, I went to my signature move. That's when I roll my knuckles across her g-spot. Back and forth slowly. It doesn't take much. Women tell me that when I do that, that is the moment that they become addicted to being fisted. Some speak in tongues. Some see dead relatives. I think Brenda was still speaking English, but it was indecipherable.

Knuckles are very hard and can make a girl sore pretty quick. A session only last a few minutes really. I slowly pulled my hand out. Leaned over and kissed her pussy lovingly before I reached for a towel. I watched her eyes. Her eyes were fixed on mine, watching to see if I was going to do anything else to her. Instead, I laid down next to her and kissed her cheek.

"Good girl," I moaned softly into her ear.

The emotional release came from that. "Thank you," she whispered. I could see the tears, but she fought them back. I used to freak out when a woman cried after she came really well. I learned that if I was doing my job, it was a very emotional thing for a woman. If I did my job well, there should always be tears. I wasn't always aiming for them. But now I knew they were a good sign.

She clutched me tightly to hide the tears. But I could feel her body shuddering. I held her tighter when I felt that.

"I don't know why I'm crying," she said. "I never cry after sex."

I smiled and told her that I must have done a good job. She nodded.

"And oh my God! I can't believe how much squirt there is!" she said.

I snickered the snicker of a confident man. "You've only been here an hour. What are we going to do the rest of the weekend?"

"Eat chili?" she replied.

I laughed. "Yes! Let's go get some chili!"

We ate and talked a little, but not much. I think I got all the energy she had. Full bellies, we went to sleep happy.

The rest of the weekend, we made huge puddles everywhere in my apartment. I went through an entire package of puppy pads by Saturday afternoon and had to hit the grocery store for more. There was plenty of fisting too. She had brought some big toys and we played with those a little. But they were rather boring after I fisted her. I swear. That might be the sorest I have ever made a pussy. She kept asking for more though. What was I to do?

After she went home, we stayed in touch. She called every once in a while. Mostly boo-hooing that the guy she was dating wouldn't fist her right or that the guy she brought home freaked out at her toy collection. In their defense, she did have some monster toys that could be a little intimidating.

When she started dating Ben, she knew he was a keeper. Her kink and his kink were a perfect match. She called me and made small talk, gradually getting around to the real reason she called.

"Will you tell him how to do that thing with your knuckles?"

I laughed. "Sure. Put him on the phone."

Ben and I talked a little. Yes, I explained my little trick and they hung up happy.

So, there I was, making dinner. I see the caller ID and it said Minnesota. I smiled and answered.

"Hello Brenda," I greeted. "Long time, no call."

"Hello," she answered. "I need your help."

"No how ya doing? No, How's Chicago? Just get right to it, huh?"

She laughed. "Ben is coming home from Iraq in two hours and I want to do something special for him. Got any ideas? Something really unusual maybe?"

Let me digress for a minute. Heard any good jokes lately?

A man is sitting on a train across from a busty blonde wearing a tiny miniskirt. He can't help but notice that she is not wearing panties. Despite his efforts, he is unable to stop staring. The blonde realizes he is staring and inquires, "Are you looking at my pussy?"

"Yes, I'm sorry," replies the man and promises to stop.

"It's quite all right," replies the woman, "It's actually very talented. Watch this. I'll make it blow you a kiss."

Sure enough the pussy blows him a kiss. The man, who is completely amazed, asks what else the talented pussy can do.

"I can also make it wink," says the woman. The man stares in amazement as the pussy winks at him.

"Come and sit next to me," suggests the woman, patting the seat. The man moves over and is asked, "Would you like to stick a couple of fingers in?"

Stunned, the man replies, "Good grief! Can it whistle too?!?!"

Okay. So I had just read that joke a little while before I started making dinner. It's an old joke. I had heard it a few times before. But this time, it had me giggling just like I was hearing it for the first time. And then Brenda called.

"Something unusual, huh?" I confirmed.

"Yeah. Got any ideas?"

"I do. Let's teach your pussy to whistle."

There was silence on the other end of the call for maybe a minute before she busted out laughing. And I mean, she completely lost it. It took a full two minutes before I could go on.

"Actual whistling might be a challenge. I'm not sure we can really do that. Not in two hours anyway. I'm confident. But that might take some time."

"Yeah, I didn't think you were serious."

"Oh, I'm serious. I just think actual whistling will take more than two hours. Do you have a kazoo?"

Her laughter stopped dead for a minute… And then it resumed harder than ever. I waited patiently. I wasn't the one on a deadline. Ladies, just to be honest, I have never taught a pussy a whistle. In theory though, it is very possible. If you know how a reed instrument works, you know what I mean. Performing a concerto is probably a stretch. But being able to make sound is very doable.

Anyway. She finally quit laughing after a couple minutes. And then she started again. And finally she stopped enough I could explain further.

"Are you done?" I asked seriously. As I said, I was making dinner. At this point, I was chopping vegetables for a salad.

"Yes," she giggled. But no, she wasn't quite done. She couldn't stop laughing. I continued waiting.

When she seemed to be getting it out of her system, I asked her, "Seriously. Do you have a kazoo?" That question started the whole cycle again. I understood how funny this probably sounded to her. I really did get it. But dammit, she was on a deadline and we had work to do.

"I'm serious," I told her.

"No you're not," she answered.

"I am." I told her very matter-of-factly. "You wanted to do something that is special. What is more special than a musical pussy greeting him when he comes through the door?"

I guess the visual of that was too much for her and there she was laughing uncontrollably again. This time it took another two minutes. I remained stoic, waiting for it to pass. "We're wasting time, ya know. You're down to one hour and forty five minutes."

"Okay, okay," she answered as she tried to again control of herself. "Yes, I have a kazoo. Well, my kids have a kazoo. Shall I get it?"

"Yes," i answered with all the seriousness I could muster. Now that it seemed like we might actually do this, I was starting to feel the laughter coming up. I held it in though. "You're also going to need a bicycle pump and a small vibrator."

"Oh shit, what the hell?!?!" she hollered as it sounded like she was running through her house, like rounding up the items for a crazy scavenger hunt. After a few minutes, out of breath, she said, "Okay. Now what.

"Are ya naked yet?" I asked.

"No. Where should we do this?"

"I'm thinking on the couch so that he sees you first thing when he walks in."

"Oh my God. You really are nuts, ya know!"

"So I've been told. But, you wanted something special."

A moment later, she said she was naked and sitting on the couch with the items I had her collect.

"Brenda, I remember your pussy. I remember that from all the Kegels that you do, that your pussy has AMAZING elasticity. Do you still do all those Kegels?"

"Yeah."

"You can stretch wide for fists and huge toys, but you can also shut that thing down very tight. Still true?"

"Yeah."

"Good. Get comfortable on the couch."

She did.

"Now, I want you to use the pump to fill your pussy with air."

"Oh my God," she muttered and started laughing again. There was rustling on the phone for a few seconds. And then, I heard the bicycle pump being pumped. "Shit! That feels weird."

"You can start a new fetish later. Some people are into that."

She laughed a little and I heard the sound I was waiting for. A queef, or quif, or pussy fart to those less cultured "You sound full. Good. Fill it up as much as you can."

"I have an air compressor. That might work better," she suggested.

There was a moment when I considered letting her learn a painful lesson the hard way. Ladies, an air compressor sends a tremendous amount of air into your vagina suddenly. It is impossible to control inflating yourself to ONLY your limit and it is possible to do serious damage. Just letting you know. Just for a second, I considered letting her discover this. I wondered what my legal liability might be if I let her use the air compressor and it went painfully sideways. In my head, I weighed the possibilities of air embolisms and… Well… An exploding vagina. Yes, I thought about the prospects of an exploding vagina, which the WORDS sound hilarious, but the visual does not. And then I remembered that I actually care about human beings. I'm all love and zen and whatnot, and truly want people to have a happy and healthy sex life. Serious injury is counter to that mission. Knowingly allowing someone to hurt themselves would ruin my credibility. "No. That's a bad idea. Slow and steady wins the race. Brenda, promise me that if you ever do this again, that you won't use the air compressor."

"Okay," she promised and I could hear the tire pump again.

"You don't want to cause any pain. But, you want to fill yourself up as much as you can."

"I am," she answered. "God this feels so weird."

I told her, "When you're full and you don't think you can pump any more air inside, gently remove the pump."

She giggled, "I can't believe I am doing this!" And I heard a very loud pussy fart. A mega queef, so to speak, which started her laughing again. When she started laughing, she lost all the rest of the air in one loud, long queef.

"You have to keep the air inside. So, stop laughing."

And as anyone who had been laughing and couldn't stop knows, telling you to stop laughing only makes it worse. And, she got worse. I waited again, although this was starting to wear me down and start me laughing. I heard her pumping again. And then I heard her laughing uncontrollably and heard her pussy farting just as uncontrollably. Queef, queef, queef.

"I'm sorry. I can't help it. I know where you're going with this and I can't believe we are doing this."

In spite of the laughter, which I was joining her in by this time, she managed to get herself full and hold it.

"Okay. put the kazoo right up to the hole and blow as hard as you can."

Accompanied by more laughter, I heard the music I was hoping for. If you simply blow through a kazoo or any similar mirlitons, it won't make much of a sound. And, the little bit of a sound it makes won't be much like the sound you expect. Air alone will only slightly vibrate the wax paper resonator inside. For a kazoo to sound like a kazoo, you need to hum through it. In this case, the pussy farts substituted for that humming action, combined with the air coming out, and I heard a very clear kazoo for about 5 seconds as her vaginal cavity deflated.

This sent both of us over the edge and we both had a hard time stopping our laughter. She did it again, and again we died laughing. When we managed to control it, I gave her the next instructions. "Now, we're going to play a song."

I couldn't even say that without laughing uncontrollably. It took me three attempts to say it. And then, it took her a full five minutes to stop laughing enough to inflate herself again. We were down to 45 minutes before Ben arrived.

"Okay, you're going to need both hands for this. Hold the kazoo in one hand, and as you push the air out, move the vibrator along the kazoo to see what sounds it makes.

It took about 3-4 minutes to inflate herself each time, and that's if she didn't lose it. Several times, she did. Gradually, we found that by moving the vibrator to different places on the kazoo, we could get three distinct notes. Ta-DA-taaaaahhh.

We were down to about 3 minutes. "How likely is it he'll be late"

"Ha! Not by a second!" she answered and I could hear her start to inflate.

"Leave the phone nearby. I want to hear this."

And as if on cue, I heard the commotion of him coming into the house.

"Stay there," she told him, laughing, and I heard the three notes we had discovered.

"What the-" I heard him yell. Followed by, "Do that again!" followed by hysterical laughter.

"It takes a couple minutes," she told him. I could hear her inflating again. "Here. Say hello to the fisting guy. He taught me how to do this."

Before he picked the phone up, I heard him tell her, "That guy ain't right!" And then, "Hello? Dude, what the hell?!?! You are NOT right!!" followed by more laughing by both of us as Brenda let loose with her three notes again. That had all three of us laughing so hard, we were having trouble breathing.

Brenda thanked me and hung up. I'm guessing they went to do something else with her vagina.

I got a text a couple days later telling me that she and Ben had not stopped laughing. She also asked if there are any long term health effects of doing this. All I could think of was, 'Hmmm… I wonder if she had even washed the needle on the bicycle pump before she began sticking it into her cavernous vagina.' I think she got it out of the garage, where it had probably been for years. EEEWWWW!! I didn't say anything about that. "Not that I'm aware of, as long as you don't do it to the point of pain." I mean, she was used to shoving fists and enormous toys in there. Maybe ten or fifteen years she had been doing that. I doubt some inflation was any worse. I mean, every woman has had a queef or two where a lot of air got inside when she was using her vagina. Pushing a little air inside via the tire pump is probably harmless. I honestly don't know though. I didn't tell her that either.

Ladies, if you want your pussy to whistle, I still think it is theoretically possible. I'm not entirely sure how. But thinking of how reed instruments work, I'm thinking it should be possible to craft a reed of some kind that will produce a whistle. Keep practicing and let me know if you figure anything out. Do not use an air compressor!! I may not think a tire pump will cause an exploding vagina situation, but I can see that an air compressor might. Jus' sayin'. Thank me later.

I am also hopeful one of you will experiment with a horn of some kind. It takes more air and more force behind that air to blow a horn. You could pull a muscle of some kind. But still, I am certain, technically possible. I am waiting for the day that I answer the phone and I hear a tuba. :)))))

Postscipt

The night this happened, I got a text message from a woman who asked me, "Whatcha doin'?"

I replied, "Just taught a woman to play the kazoo... With her pussy!"

"Oh shit!" she answered. "You get weirder and weirder every time I talk to you."

And after about an hour or so, I got, "I don't have a kazoo, but I have a flute."

Well, that had me laughing, literally, LOLing. I'm sure my friend on the other end of was LOLing too.

That night, I had a dream about her and that flute. I was watching TV, in the dream that is. Some kind of late night show, like The Tonight Show. The one that has car karaoke, whichever one that is. I can't tell anymore with those shows since Letterman retired. Anyway. The host introduced Celine Dion, who was on the stage about to sing her big hit from Titanic. But before she could get started, the host said, "But wait! We have a special guest!"

Well, out of the wings, here comes my friend with her flute. With her hair and makeup looking spectacular for TV, she was wearing a beautiful dress and a big smile. The crowd erupted in wild applause. Celine Dion gave her a hug like an old friend and resumed her position at the microphone. My friend hiked up her dress around her waist and plopped up on a bar stool next to her. And together, they did a passionate duet of the famous song with my friend as the queefing flautist.

Afterwards, the crowd went crazy. She hopped off the stool, allowing her dress to fall down. They both took a bow hand-in-hand. Celine Dion gave my friend another hug that, to me, seemed a little long and creepy. The host came over and gave her a hug that, to me, also seemed a little long and creepy. Members of the band were coming over giving her long, creepy hugs. The crowd was so frenzied that the host had to shout as he thanked them for their performance. End of show and end of dream.

Yeah, maybe she's right. I just get weirder and weirder.

www.ingramcontent.com/pod-product-compliance
Lightning Source LLC
Chambersburg PA
CBHW051133250726

48655CB00007B/3041